I0791758

SKINNY *Myths*

UNPLUG FROM THE LIES

Laina Joseph

BALBOA.PRESS

A DIVISION OF HAY HOUSE

Balboa Press books may be ordered through booksellers or by contacting:

Balboa Press
A Division of Hay House
1663 Liberty Drive
Bloomington, IN 47403
www.balboapress.com
1 (877) 407-4847

Print information available on the last page.

ISBN: 978-1-9822-4706-5 (sc)
ISBN: 978-1-9822-4707-2 (e)

Library of Congress Control Number: 2020908173

Balboa Press rev. date: 05/13/2020

CONTENTS

DEDICATION

To my dad, thank you for being my first editor. Even though you are no longer here, I know that you are proud of my accomplishments. And to my husband, Duane, thank you for your unwavering love and support and always being my number one fan.

INTRODUCTION

I have been struggling with my weight since I was ten. I have tried so many different diets and exercise programs that I made myself crazy. I have cried over my weight and blamed it for many situations in my life that weren't going my way. Now, finally I have triumphed, overcome! Yay! I am definitely not skinny but I am at a healthy weight, have excess energy and found an eating plan that works for me. So, the story should be over, right? I should be living happily ever after in a bikini on a beach somewhere with a fruit smoothie and sunscreen. Unfortunately, that is just not the case.

Losing weight has been a process and a journey. I was under the assumption that losing weight would solve a good majority of my problems but I was wrong. I was living with mistaken myths that once I lost weight my life would look a particular way. What is even worse is that I realized that if I had confronted, examined and resolved these myths before I lost the weight, I wouldn't have struggled all these years with my image and self esteem. I had to learn it the hard way. I'm still learning because it's a process.

I am now on a new journey with my body in learning how to maintain my weight. The sad thing is weight maintenance can be just as difficult as weight loss! I wrote these myths down to remind myself of the new person, mentally, physically and emotionally that I have created myself to be. I hope it also helps you on your journey.

The book is set up to be thought provoking and provide places to journal your thoughts. It is time for you to detect the lies and become your own myth-buster!

1

You'll Be Happy

I always thought I would be happy when the scale reached a particular number. The funny thing is that even when I achieved that goal, I still wasn't happy. Now that I am at my goal weight range, I'm ecstatic! Not because I reached the goal but simply because I choose to be.

Reality: Being happy just requires you to be happy.

They say a picture is worth a thousand words.
Draw, doodle, or add pictures to envision the life you want in this area.

Take on choosing to be happy moment by moment. You can start with the little things that you are grateful for, like savoring your first cup of morning coffee. (I don't drink coffee but everyone who does always look so happy to have that first cup!)

It is important to note that we as human beings have access to a range of emotions to express ourselves. We should experience them all as appropriate. All I am saying is what would your life look like if your predominant emotion was to be happy, instead of sad, or angry? Or any other emotion?

Write a list of 5 things that you are grateful for or that make you happy.

____

____

____

____

____

____

____

____

____

____

____

____

____

____

You'll Find Love

I thought that once I reached my ideal weight that I would instantaneously meet the man of my dreams. He would think that I was amazing and we would get married. Very childish, I know, and unfortunately it was very true for me.

Reality: Men and whether or not they treat you well have nothing to do with your weight.

I had to realize that I had collapsed the feelings of losing weight and finding love together and as long I was overweight, I was programming myself to not find love.

They say a picture is worth a thousand words.
Draw, doodle, or add pictures to envision the life you want in this area.

Have you collapsed your love life and weight loss together?

If so, start noticing those thoughts that defeat you. For example, thoughts such as nobody is ever going to love me like this. Write those thoughts down and ask yourself if they are really true and challenge them. If a friend said that to you, what would you say to him or her?

How can you love and appreciate yourself as you are right now? What action steps can you take towards finding the relationship of your dreams? Write them down.

3 | You'll Be Rich

I know there is no basis for this, but I just have this image of myself at my ideal weight and I am always rich in my imagination.

Reality: Weight and money were two other worlds that I had collapsed together along with finding my dream man! Acquiring wealth requires a certain amount of patience, knowledge, action steps and persistence. It has nothing to do with weight except that weight loss also requires a certain amount of patience, knowledge, action steps and persistence.

They say a picture is worth a thousand words.
Draw, doodle, or add pictures to envision the life you want in this area.

Have you collapsed your finances and weight loss together?

If so, notice what thoughts you have to say about weight and money. Mine were, if I was rich, I could hire a personal chef and trainer. Even better, rich men only date skinny women. Write those thoughts down and challenge each one.

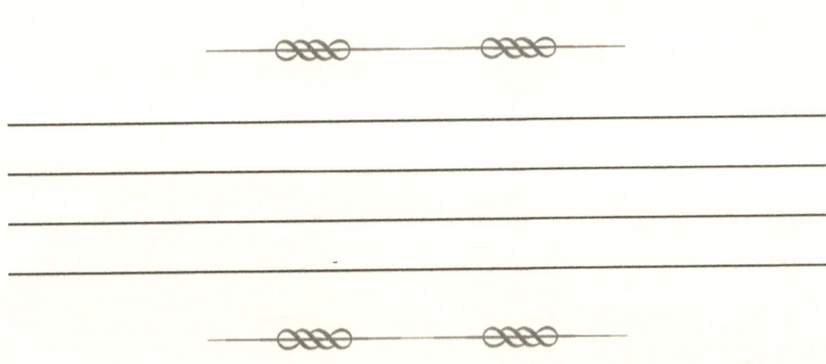

Is your weight affecting your energy level such that it affects your productivity? Is there a health concern and/or medical bills that need to be taken into consideration that adversely affect your health and finances? If so, this can serve as motivation to stay healthy.

What are some successful steps you have taken for weight loss? How can those steps be used for acquiring wealth? Or vice versa?

4 | *Your Clothes Will Fit Better*

I used to think that certain clothes didn't look good on me because I was overweight. I figured nothing would look good on me except baggy clothes so I was waiting to get to my ideal weight to express my style and feel good in clothes.

Reality: How well clothes fit is based on body shape, height and tailoring. Odds are certain styles that didn't look good on you when you were heavy may still not bring out your best features. Most fashionistas will tell you that those who look amazing in clothes get them tailored to fit their body and wear the proper undergarments to create the perfect look.

They say a picture is worth a thousand words.
Draw, doodle, or add pictures to envision the life you want in this area.

How well do your clothes fit you? Too baggy? Too tight? Do they flatter your figure and reflect your personal sense of style?

If you can't be objective about how you look, get a friend who has great style to give you some pointers. Go through your wardrobe and get rid of clothes that no longer fit your new image and that don't make you feel good.

5 | *You'll Be Considered More Attractive*

I considered myself to be the ugly duckling growing up. One of the reasons that I was straight A student in school was because I knew I wasn't going to get by on my looks! As I have gotten older, I have gotten better looking, no more braces, acne, or crazy looking hair. I have also grown more comfortable in my own skin and in my natural abilities. Still, I always wanted to be that girl that had men falling all over her! In my mind that girl was thin.

Reality: Society puts forth impossible beauty standards to live up to. It takes a team of people to create the images we see on television and in magazines. In their world, skinny is a component to being beautiful. However, the most important person who determines how attractive you are is you. It's like a Jedi mind trick: if you say you are gorgeous, then guess what! You are! If you say you're not, then you're not. Besides, nothing can truly account for why one person is attracted to another; it's chemistry.

They say a picture is worth a thousand words.
Draw, doodle, or add pictures to envision the life you want in this area.

How attractive do you consider yourself? Do they change according to what kind of day you are having? How do you feel about your clothes, hair and makeup? Does it reflect your inner self?

Once again, if you can't be objective, get a good friend to go through this process with you. Take a look at the type of women you whose style you admire and see if you can incorporate that style into your own. If it is time for some updating, go out and get that hair appointment, make-up consultation and new wardrobe. (Just make sure you are responsible with the budget!)

6 | *People Will Treat You Better/Be Nicer to You*

I used to think that people would treat me better if I were thin. I was pretty much a people pleaser and I always wanted everybody else to be happy. The problem was that I wasn't. I accepted unacceptable behavior in my relationships and got taken advantage of.

Reality: You teach people how to treat you. You are now a newer, classier, sexier model. Make them treat you accordingly.

They say a picture is worth a thousand words.
Draw, doodle, or add pictures to envision the life you want in this area.

Changing relationship dynamics that are already entrenched can be difficult. I started by checking in with myself first. I asked myself, how do I feel about this? Then I addressed the situation with that individual, usually on a time delay because I truly needed to sort out my feelings. As I got more comfortable, the time delay got much shorter.

Being treated in a particular fashion is really about creating acceptable boundaries. Do you have relationships that you feel don't honor you as a person?

Could an aspect of that relationship be changed? Are you willing to address the issue in order to move forward?

7   *You'll Have the Perfect Body*

I thought that once I reached my ideal weight, I would have the perfect body.

Reality: Even models' bodies aren't perfect. Their photographs get airbrushed and photoshopped. Also losing weight doesn't necessarily shape and tone your body. Muscle and strength training are needed in order to effect body shape within the parameters of your given body type and genetic make up.

They say a picture is worth a thousand words.
Draw, doodle, or add pictures to envision the life you want in this area.

Now that you've lost weight, are there still areas of your body that you are unhappy with? Could this be resolved through specific exercises? If not, is plastic surgery necessary? (This may be the case if you lost weight very rapidly.) Consider making peace with all the imperfect areas of your body and love it anyway. If you can't, make a plan to fix it. List your action plan below.

8 Your Feet Will Shrink

I was excited at the prospect of wearing a smaller size shoe because it always seemed like those shoes had more selections on sale!

Reality: Some people's feet may shrink but yours may not.

They say a picture is worth a thousand words.
Draw, doodle, or add pictures to envision the life you want in this area.

Try different shoes on anyway! You may find new styles or that you are able to wear different heel lengths because it is easier to support your body weight. What new styles are you willing to try that reflect your new lifestyle?

9 Your Calves Will Shrink

I thought that when you lost weight, you'd lose it all over but for some reason my calves are still very large. So large that I can't wear the knee-high boots that create such a sophisticated look to an outfit. I have found this development to be very disappointing. I also have that same issue with my arms. Same concept, different body part.

Reality: You can't spot reduce.

They say a picture is worth a thousand words.
Draw, doodle, or add pictures to envision the life you want in this area.

There are specific exercises to define and tone calves. There are also boots that are made for wider calves. You can also get your boots altered to fit you. Also, make peace with your legs. What's your plan to showcase your sexy legs?

10 — Your Chest, Butt and Thighs Unfortunately May Shrink

I enjoy my new body but I am not exactly enjoying the shrinkage of some of my more celebrated parts. It can be a little shocking to go down a bra cup size or become less of a curvy woman. If you tie your weight in with your identity, you may have to mourn the loss of the former woman you created yourself to be.

Reality: Losing weight transforms your entire body, not just the parts you don't like.

They say a picture is worth a thousand words.
Draw, doodle, or add pictures to envision the life you want in this area.

Be open to accepting the new you and work on accentuating what works for you now. More than likely you still have curves, just less of them. Find fun ways to play them up! List them here.

11   *You'll Love Your New Face*

As I was losing weight, I could see the change instantly in my face even if it wasn't directly reflected in the rest of my body. Sometimes I felt like I was looking at a stranger in the mirror.

Reality: As much as we say we want to, change can be scary or unnerving because it threatens your identity.

They say a picture is worth a thousand words.
Draw, doodle, or add pictures to envision the life you want in this area.

The person in the mirror doesn't have to be a stranger. Look at yourself often in the mirror to get accustomed to your new face. What do you like about it? What's your best feature? Is it more pronounced now that you have lost weight? Take time to play with different make-up looks to find ways to maximize your best features. Make your action plan below.

12 · You've Completely Resolved All the Issues that Caused You to Gain Weight in the First Place

A co-worker once commented to me that she didn't understand how people could become obese. I told her that we all deal with issues differently and that weight gain may be a physical manifestation of them or maybe they have other health issues that affect their weight.

Reality: Let's forget about other people. Only you know why you gained weight and only you know why you were able to lose it.

They say a picture is worth a thousand words.
Draw, doodle, or add pictures to envision the life you want in this area.

If you've lost weight, then you were able to deal with some or all key issues. To ensure continued success, write down your trigger issues, situations and foods. For each item, create a strategy or multiple strategies to address it. For example, I tend to overeat when I am anxious. Now when I find myself overeating for no reason, I ask myself what am I anxious or worried about. Once I can identify the cause of the emotion, I am able to address that issue instead of sabotaging myself.

You may need or want to seek additional help/therapy to address some of these issues and/or situations. It is also important to keep in mind that the issues caused by the weight gain are probably affecting you in other areas of your life. Be responsible to yourself and get additional help if you need it. You probably didn't of your weight overnight and it may take time to resolve underlying issues even after you've lost the weight. If you could wave a magic wand, what are some of the core issues around weight loss that could be resolved overnight? List them here.

____

____

____

____

____

____

____

____

____

13 Your Cellulite Will Magically Disappear

From time to time I consider my cellulite. I don't know why; it's not hurting anybody. However, I do feel that it would be nice for cellulite to go its own separate way. When I do break down and buy a cream or lotion, it usually says something like reduced weight often reduces the look of cellulite.

Reality: No matter what your size, cellulite is very difficult to get rid of.

They say a picture is worth a thousand words.
Draw, doodle, or add pictures to envision the life you want in this area.

Do you really want to take on the cellulite battle? If so, there are creams, potions and treatments for that. If not, do what I do and pretend it is not even there! What's your cellulite action plan?

14 You'll Wear Daring, Sexier Clothes

Actually, I do wear sexier clothes. Or maybe I feel sexier because I now wear clothes that flatter my shape and my body type! However, there are some outfits hanging in my closet that even I am a little too shy to wear. Besides, the point is to find a look or style that complements not only your personality but also the occasion. The more comfortable you are in your clothes, the more self confident you will be and that is very sexy.

Reality: Weight loss doesn't mean that you are instantly going to be transformed into a sex kitten overnight, unless of course, you want to!

They say a picture is worth a thousand words.
Draw, doodle, or add pictures to envision the life you want in this area.

If you feel good in sexier clothes, by all means wear them! If you want to wear these clothes, but you are too shy, work on the shyness first and take baby steps. You may want to update your lingerie. Nobody else might see it but you know it's there. How many different ways can you express your sexy, flirty self?

15 | *You'll Be More Self Confident/Outgoing*

I was never one to truly live life on the sidelines but I wasn't exactly playing full out either. When I lost weight, I thought I would have a personality transplant and be the life of the party.

Reality: Unless you make a conscious decision to do so, your overall temperament and personality will stay the same. However, weight loss may lift some of the social/emotional barriers that stop you from expressing yourself fully.

They say a picture is worth a thousand words.
Draw, doodle, or add pictures to envision the life you want in this area.

If you are self-confident and outgoing, great! Continue as you are. If not, practice faking it until you make it. Pick someone who is extremely confident to emulate. Ask yourself what would they do, feel, wear, say and act in any given situation. Then go do it! List some action steps here.

16 | *You'll Be Healthy*

Since I was about 10, I've hated going to the doctor because the doctor would inevitably turn to my mother and tell her that I need to lose weight. Yet, outside that one factor, I was always healthy.

Reality: Yes, weight is a factor in your picture of overall health and weight loss can dramatically improve the odds of staving off serious illnesses. However, being overweight does not necessarily mean that you are not healthy and being skinny does not necessarily mean that you are healthy.

They say a picture is worth a thousand words.
Draw, doodle, or add pictures to envision the life you want in this area.

Get check ups on a regular basis to make sure that you are healthy and if you need to make changes, do it. Know your health history and don't buy into scare tactics about your body. Make a list of the healthy habits that already are part of your lifestyle. List any lingering issues and possible ways to deal with them.

17   *You Won't Have to Exercise as Much*

How I wish that was true! Generally, I am at the gym 4-5 days a week more or less depending on my schedule. I have found for myself personally, that an exercise regimen keeps my mind and body focused on my fitness goals. When I stop going to the gym, I lose my focus and gain weight. I exercise just as much or even harder to maintain my new lower weight.

Reality: Exercise is an integral part of weight loss and maintenance. You may not exercise the same way during your weight loss phase as maintenance, but finding a way to stay active creates a healthy lifestyle and all its associated benefits.

They say a picture is worth a thousand words.
Draw, doodle, or add pictures to envision the life you want in this area.

You may want to consider talking to a personal trainer about new exercise goals and the best way to maintain your weight loss. This would be a great way to address those stubborn areas that you are still struggling with. How active are you? Are you happy with your overall level of fitness? Now that you have lost the weight, have you slacked off?

18 · You Can Eat Whatever You Want, When You Want

I like to eat because I enjoy it and I hate to deny myself. Sometimes it may seem like thin people eat what they want, whenever they want. Upon closer inspection, I have noticed that they usually have found a way to compensate for the extra calories that they are taking in. They either eat less that day or they work extra hard at the gym. Since we don't see what they do 24 hours a day, it took me awhile to realize that they truly do account for what they eat. Some people are just genetically blessed.

Reality: Eating whatever you wanted probably led to you being overweight in the first place! When talking about weight loss, people always mention that you should be focused on changing your lifestyle. It can be difficult to deprive yourself of particular foods and make the change permanent. It's more important to put your life in balance so that you can enjoy food and your ideal body.

They say a picture is worth a thousand words.
Draw, doodle, or add pictures to envision the life you want in this area.

Since you worked so hard to lose the weight, don't blow it! As you adjust to maintaining your desired weight, continue to monitor your foods and exercise. It's all about finding the balance between your lifestyle and your optimum weight. You may still need to avoid certain foods until you can handle it. List 5 trigger foods here.

19 | *All Your Friends, Family and Loved Ones Support Your New Self*

Food is central to how I socialize. I like to go out to eat and enjoy great conversation along with great food. When I started my weight loss process, I sometimes made the choice not to go out with certain people because of the bad food choices they made. I knew I would be tempted to eat the wrong thing and often I did. I felt like I was missing out. Now I plan ahead to order something appropriate and I look forward to eating that meal! For new restaurants, I look up menus ahead of time and figure out at least two choices that I would like to order. It doesn't always have to be a salad! The other thing I realized is that more often than not, the person I was eating with didn't have the type of body that I was striving for.

I also have friends who like to feed me. Don't get me wrong I appreciate that. However, they wanted me to eat food that was not conducive to weight loss. I learned the art of saying no, repeatedly even though there was a part of me that felt guilty. It was more important to stand up for the new body I was creating.

Reality: Change can be difficult for those around you as well as for yourself. They like you the way you are and are comfortable with it. Friends and family may unwittingly sabotage your efforts for weight loss. Sometimes, they have a vested interest in keeping you the way you are. Take 100% responsibility for your body and don't let anyone impede your efforts.

They say a picture is worth a thousand words.
Draw, doodle, or add pictures to envision the life you want in this area.

Identify situations and people that may sabotage your weight loss/ maintenance efforts. List them here and for each situation write down a possible action to take. You may not always follow through on your actions all the time! That's okay. Use the information as feedback to prepare you for the next time. For example, I always give myself three dining options from the menu and label them from healthiest to the least healthy option. That way I don't feel pressured to always eat salad.

20 | *Just Because You Think You Are Skinny Doesn't Mean that Everybody Thinks So*

You've worked hard on your weight loss and you're feeling great. I noticed something interesting among 2 sets of friends. One set would say, "You're getting too skinny; you should stop." The other set would say, "Wow, you look great; you're almost there. Keep up the good work." I felt confused and sometimes annoyed. Since I had been on this weight loss roller coaster for most of my life, I had a set number in my head of what my ideal weight should be from doctors, nutritionists and other diet programs I had done. I had to come to my own personal truth about the range in which I felt healthy and capable of maintaining that weight.

Reality: Only you know an appropriate, realistic weight for your lifestyle, unless a doctor tells you otherwise. You have to take into consideration diet, frequency of exercise, muscle mass, stress and other lifestyle factors that affect your overall health.

They say a picture is worth a thousand words.
Draw, doodle, or add pictures to envision the life you want in this area.

Evaluate your weight loss and maintenance goals. If you don't have any, create one or two. You may want to talk to your doctor and a personal trainer to get professional opinions. Given your lifestyle, what works for you? What are some challenge areas? For example, for me vacations are a huge challenge because I want to eat everything and I don't get to exercise as much!

21 | *You Will Not Be Judged as Harshly Being Skinny*

I have found that most people still make comments about heavy people and feel justified in thinking that something is wrong with the person. They don't mind telling you, now that you've lost weight, because they think that you will agree. I do still get angry with people who are so critical, clueless and insensitive. I usually challenge their comments and other times I just shake my head and can't be bothered.

Reality: People can be very judgmental and you yourself may be one of them! Just keep in mind that if they are judgmental about weight, then they are judgmental about other things as well.

They say a picture is worth a thousand words.
Draw, doodle, or add pictures to envision the life you want in this area.

If you are around people who are constantly making comments that bother you, you may want to consider not associating with those people as much. Still wanna be friends? Explain to them how those statements make you feel. You may have to do this more than once. Just be consistent and they'll get the message. Remember, what they say reflects their issues, not yours! Write out what you could possibly say to them below.

22   *People Will Like You More/ You'll Like People More*

Part of losing weight for me is dealing with self acceptance. Sometimes it is easier to be a normal weight and blend in. Other times, even if you have lost the weight, you still feel alone amongst a crowd. I thought that as I accepted myself more that I would like more people and become more acceptable of them. What I realized is that I can be picky! I either like you or I don't. The only difference is that now, I don't take not getting along with someone personally. I don't worry about other people accepting me, I just worry about how I feel about me!

Reality: People get along for lots of different reasons. Weight can be a reason to bond with someone else because you have similar experiences and struggles. However, a lot of other factors go into creating quality relationships.

They say a picture is worth a thousand words.
Draw, doodle, or add pictures to envision the life you want in this area.

Are you a people pleaser? What are its advantages and disadvantages? List them. Practice listening to your inner guidance and start saying no to situations and people that don't support you.

23   *You Are Taken Less Seriously/More Seriously*

It is interesting because as I have lost weight, I have had to make requests and really be honest to myself about taking caring of my body and my health. Every time someone tried to sabotage me, I found myself getting angry. It was as if to say, these people didn't believe me. Considering that I eventually give in, they were right. It made me stand my ground even stronger. I had to stay focused on my goal of achieving a healthy lifestyle.

Also, there is a dynamic of losing weight that made me feel smaller. I'm short so one of my fears on losing weight was that people would belittle my presence and what I have to say.

Reality: It takes some time for people to adjust to the new you and the fact that you are serious about your weight loss results. They are not trying to take you less seriously consciously but old habits die hard. You are the one making the change, not them, so you are the one who has to stand your ground.

They say a picture is worth a thousand words.
Draw, doodle, or add pictures to envision the life you want in this area.

In terms of losing presence, there are many short, thin people who have an amazing presence. Having a presence requires you to be true to yourself and have the confidence to express it.

Consider that in the area of weight loss, friends and family may not take you seriously because you have been on this particular merry go round for a long time. For many of us, years! As you take the actions that are consistent with a person who is serious about their health and weight, they will eventually come to respect your actions. Don't worry about them, worry about you! What are some ways that you express your authentic self?

24 · *People Will No Longer Give You Advice about Your Weight*

From the time I started gaining weight as a teenager, my weight seemed to be an open commentary amongst family. Oh, you've gained weight or oh, you've lost weight and then we go into the latest exercise and diet plan. I always felt like there was an undertone that something was either wrong with me or us (if we both happen to be overweight). This time around, a close friend of mine commented negatively on what I was doing. I stopped talking to her about it completely and only talked to people who I knew could support me the way I needed to be supported.

Reality: Weight loss is a topic about which people always have something to say. The main goal here is that as you stop talking about weight issues, so will they. Even if they do, you can always redirect the conversation onto something else if you want to.

They say a picture is worth a thousand words.
Draw, doodle, or add pictures to envision the life you want in this area.

Reclaim your body image for yourself. Identify the people in your life that you talk about weight with. Look at each name. Are they helping or hurting the situation? Decide how you need to be supported and request specific help. If you feel that you can't talk to certain people about your weight loss experience then don't.

25 | *The Voice in Your Head that Tells You that You Are Fat Will Go Away Automatically*

I was looking in the mirror the other day thinking, man, I lost all this weight, why am I still fat? Highly unenlightened thinking to say the least. I felt like I wasn't good enough and that I still had a long way to go on this weight loss journey even though I had already dropped 5 sizes! When will it end? When will whatever you are striving for be good enough? I've been working with this inner critic because it truly is counter productive to any positive strides I am making. I consider this part of my recovery process as being a perfectionist.

Reality: We all (or maybe just some!) have this inner critic that can really do a number on our self esteem and sabotage us far better than any outside source. The voice may be the voice of a parent or someone who told you that you were fat or that you would never lose weight. At some point you internalized the information and now it is taking up residence in your head and hijacking your emotions along with it. Chances are this critic has a lot of negative comments about other areas of your life too! The reality is that the inner critic is not reality!

They say a picture is worth a thousand words.
Draw, doodle, or add pictures to envision the life you want in this area.

The whole weight loss process has taught me how to be nicer to myself. I don't have to eat things that don't honor me to feel better. Honoring and expressing my feelings make me feel better.

Do you have an inner critic? If you don't, bravo! However, if you do, what does the critic have to say about your weight loss? Write it down and read it over. Is it valid or is there an underlying issue? Go through each one and debunk them. When your inner critic feels like sharing, acknowledge the thought and remind yourself that you are striving toward something else now. This is an ongoing process. Don't expect the inner critic to be gone overnight, but also don't allow it to get in the way of your dreams.

AFTERWORD

I wrote this book prior to marriage and kids. The 25 Myths were born out of an epiphany that after chasing this seemingly unattainable number on the scale, my life still had not dramatically transformed. Intuitively, I knew this not to be true, but the media messaging that beautiful, thin, rich, happy models are the standard led me to expect a fairy tale ending! This book was a wake-up call to dispel societal myths and dig deeper into what really matters. For me that was creating a life that I love.

Once married, I gained all my weight back and more! Then pregnancy came along with an additional 40 pounds and labor-induced high blood pressure. Five years later, I have lost 95 pounds and normalized my blood pressure. The more challenging and complicated life became, the more creative I needed to be about health and fitness.

After all this time, I decided to publish this book because those pesky myths are still distorting people's perceptions about health, fitness and weight loss.

ABOUT THE AUTHOR

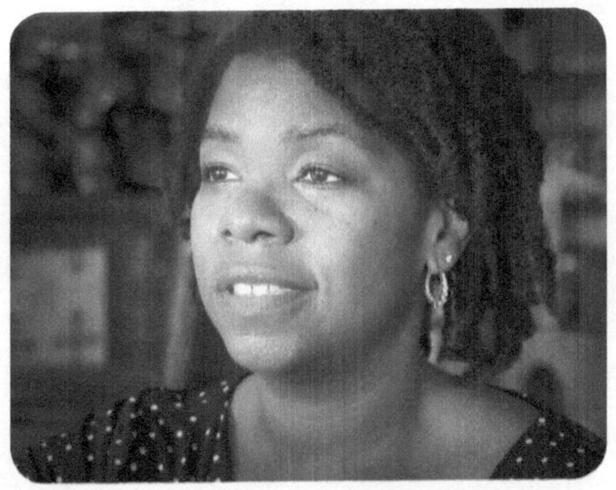

I am a writer, teacher, wife, mom, stepmom and self-avowed nerd. I am also an adventurous, part-time hobbyist who is a coach, belly dancer and Reiki Master. I believe that the title of "Mom" should be incorporated into the woman, not eclipse her. I use manifesting principles to create and transform my life. I am quirky but practical and have found navigating motherhood to be the biggest adventure of all. I am sharing my insights and journey in a blog. Come join me at:

https://thelainiway.com/

9 781982 247065